BUILDING INDESTRUCTIBLE ATHLETES

The Small Things That Make Athletes Great!

BUILDING INDESTRUCTIBLE ATHLETES

The Small Things That Make Athletes Great!

By
DONNY MATEAKI

Copyright © 2018 Donny Mateaki

Publishing Services by Happy Self Publishing
www.happyselfpublishing.com

Year: 2018

All rights reserved. No reproduction, transmission or copy of this publication can be made without the written consent of the author in accordance with the provision of the Copyright Acts. Any person doing so will be liable to civil claims and criminal prosecution.

DISCLAIMER

This publication contains the opinions and ideas of the author. It is intended to provide helpful and educational material on the subjects addressed in the publication. It is sold with the understanding that the author and publisher are not engaged in rendering medical, health or any other kind of professional services in the book. The reader should consult his or her medical, health or other competent professional before adopting any of the suggestions in this book or drawing inferences from it. The author and publisher specifically disclaim all responsibility of any liability, loss or risk, personal or otherwise which is incurred in consequence directly or indirectly of the use and the application of any of the contents of this book.

Dedication

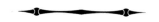

There are so many people I want to thank and dedicate this book to. First and foremost, I want to thank God. He has revealed His higher purpose for me.

To my parents, Uheina and Tele, thank you for always encouraging me and my six siblings to do our best.

To my wife, thank you for believing in me, especially in those times that I didn't believe in myself. Thank you for doing the most important work in our family; raising and educating our children. There is no way I could ever do what you do, and I am so lucky to have you in my life.

To my kids, you are my why. You are the reason I get up early, work my hardest and stay up late and do whatever it takes to provide the best I possibly can for you guys.

To my siblings, thank you for the love and support while we were kids and all the way until now. I never knew that having so many siblings was so rare, until I left home.

To my in-laws Ane & William Phillips, and my wife's siblings, thank you for taking me in and making me feel like a part of the family right away.

To my coaches and teachers that spent extra time investing in me because you saw something special, thank you! To all of my Iolani ohana--thank you for taking me in, supporting and mentoring me to become a better student, athlete and all-around person. College was a breeze because of my experience at Iolani. My high school is a special place. Not solely due to the academic excellence of the school, but because of the love and care that the teachers, counselors, coaches, and staff show the students. You are all truly remarkable.

To all of the boys from back home, and my brothers here in Seattle. You are family to me.

I would like to thank my team. Zach Foster, you are one of the best strength and conditioning coaches in the business, and we are so lucky to have you as part of the team. D'Anthony Smith, thank you for your feedback which helped us to take the next step in our business. Your advice and help are invaluable. In life, the luckiest thing that can happen, is meeting the right people. Zach and D'Anthony, you have impacted my work and personal life for the better, in so many ways.

Last but not least, I want to thank the athletes and clients that we have been given the privilege to work with currently, and in the past. You have given us the opportunity to do what we love, day in and day out-- and that is priceless. You have all helped us to grow alongside of you. We are committed to always learning and growing so you will get the best results possible.

Thank you! We are truly blessed.

Contents

Introduction 11

Eliminating Non-Contact Injuries 15

The DM Athletics Training Method 23

    Step 1: Nutrition Evaluation. 25

    Step 2: Posture Evaluation. 35

    Step 3: Mobility Screening. 45

    Step 4: Performance and Growth Tracking. 53

    Step 5: Personalized Programs. 65

    Step 6: Heart Rate Variability Monitoring. 79

    Step 7: Re Test and Modifications. 93

    Step 8 : Mindset 99

Conclusion 113

Introduction

What if I told you that there is a way to train athletes so that they not only perform their best and reach their potential, but are also made indestructible in the process? It might sound gimmicky, or like a false claim--but this is exactly what we've helped to achieve, while working with our athletes. The goal of this book is to take the performance level of athletes to their maximum potential. All while keeping them safe for as long as they play, and helping injured athletes to get back to the top of their game. The only potential injuries athletes might experience when they utilize this method, would be the result of colliding into other athletes, or the experience of other athletes falling onto them. Everything else--from non-contact ACL injuries, torn achilles, pulled hamstrings, separated shoulders, and even death during athletic competition, is completely avoided with this method.

Before sharing my method, however, I think it would be best that I familiarize you with my own personal journey in athletics. Doing so, will help you to understand why I am so passionate about training, and helping motivated individuals realize their full athletic potential.

Coming out of high school, I was a highly recruited football player, my position was Defensive End. I was offered the opportunity to play college football at several schools, but ultimately chose to play at the University of Washington. After redshirting in my first year, I went through a shoulder surgery, to repair a torn ligament. During the next season, I began starting halfway through the season, leading to a Freshman All-American honor, as well as attention from NFL coaches and teams. In the following season, however, I suffered a foot injury, which changed the trajectory of my career.

When I injured my foot, I began a training and rehabilitation program. Despite working diligently to regain my strength, movement, and athletic skill, I failed to see true improvement. As a result, my hips would overcompensate for my tight foot and ankle, whenever I did squats and lunges. I would end up seeing this play out on the field. The injury in my foot, was affecting my ability to change direction--my hips began tightening up, and I could no longer change direction like I once had. This in turn, affected me making plays which required me to change direction. With athletics, you often see this sort of domino effect. As a result of injury, one thing leads to the next, and before you know it, you're wondering how things have changed so quickly. It felt extremely frustrating to no longer able to execute the normal plays I'd easily been able to make, prior to my injury. My abilities deteriorated to the point that although I'd been a starter in my freshman season, I had to ride the bench halfway through my senior season. After I finished my Senior season, I was not given the opportunity to play in the NFL, due to my inability to change directions, loss of speed and strength. I wasn't able to accomplish my goal of playing at the highest level, and it was devastating. I was left wondering why I had gone through that experience. I knew there was a reason I'd been through that disappointment—I just didn't realize that the reason was to help others avoid the hardships I had gone through.

As the saying goes, hindsight is 20/20. Looking back at this time in my life, I see that it was a blessing. It gave me a deeper insight into the small things that I was doing, in order to get back to top performance. I consider myself to have a strong spiritual life--and in light of that lens, I believe that this experience helped me to realize that training is my calling. My purpose extends beyond making money or achieving success. It is to help others to overcome the obstacles that I myself could not overcome; but even more importantly, to help others avoid that experience altogether.

The training method that I'm about to share with you, developed as a result of pouring myself into learning and testing what actually works. There are countless philosophies and methods that promise to improve athletic performance; I've studied a lot of them and implemented them with the athletes I train. Unfortunately, most of the methods and philosophies did not produce the results they promised, especially on athletes who play at the college and professional level.

I can confidently tell you that the training method outlined below, has not only helped my clients reach the height of their athletic abilities--but it has even led many of them to play professionally, and prolong their careers. Skeptics will wonder why I'd share my method and let others in on my secrets, but in all honesty, there is no secret to training. Hard work, discipline, dedication, and focus always win out--while the method below will provide the guide to help you take the right steps at the right time, when it comes to your training program.

Eliminating Non-Contact Injuries

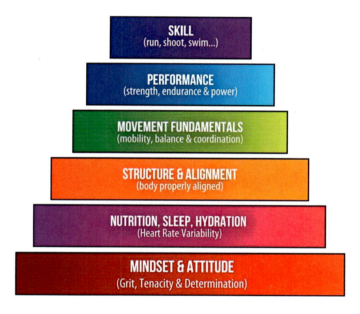

Here are the components of our training philosophy. Each one is important and they build upon each other. When one piece is not where it needs to be, the athlete will not perform at their highest level, causing injuries to incur. Mindset & Attitude is the approach that each athlete must take. Not only to competition, but to training, practice, their nutrition and every other environment which has to do with their preparation for their sport.

We do not cover the skill portion, because that is what athletes do at practice: work on their skills. Whether it be shooting a basketball, route running, hitting a ball, or mastering any other skill specific to their sport. The majority of an athlete's time is spent on mastering their skill, and the performance block of the pyramid. Here's the thing. You need more than just skill, for any given sport. Let's take basketball for example. In basketball, an athlete needs to run and play defense at a high level--not just shoot the ball well. Stephen Curry is arguably the best shooter of all time, and he is still an excellent athlete. If all he could do was shoot a basketball--but was unable to run fast, jump high, and play defense, he would not be in the NBA. The same can be said for any other athlete that is highly celebrated for a skill in their sport. You need more than just skill, to both play at your highest level and prevent getting hurt.

The one thing I found most amazing, once we pulled all of the parts of this method into place, was that there isn't a single athlete that has been with us for at least three months that have experienced any non-contact injuries during their season. Additionally, the overall injury rate of our athletes dropped by 95%. To clarify, non- contact injuries are injuries which take place when athletes change direction, jump, land, or even run. On the flip side, when there is a collision, and an athlete gets hurt, that is referred to as a contact injury. This method will not prevent contact injuries from occurring--but it will give athletes the best chance to stay healthy, even when they experience collisions.

The reason we are able to accomplish this, is because we've put all the pieces that matter, together. There are eight different components to the method, and each one is extremely important. There is no magic bullet when it comes to doing this, but rather several factors all working together, which will help you to achieve injury-free seasons for your athletes. Our sample size isn't the largest, and definitely not the smallest. Since implementing this method, we've worked with hundreds of different athletes. It's amazing that we have had zero non-contact injuries, with this varied group. We have also worked with athletes that have sustained multiple non-contact ACL injuries prior to working with us--but they too, have gone on to eliminate those issues, thereafter.

We have seen players we've helped, go on to play in the NFL, after suffering multiple ACL injuries. As the industry goes, he later decided to work with other coaches. Location and input from agents, can have an influence on where an athlete trains, and we do respect that. However, sadly, there have been some who go on to experience those injuries again. They experience another non-contact ACL, and the next thing you know, their career is in jeopardy.

This method will work, but it will not continue to work if you just all of the sudden discontinue the process, and begin working with people who do not value putting an emphasis on each one of the components. I love to lift weights and run, so when I first looked at each of the components I wasn't convinced that they were important. While playing at the high school level, I was benching over 400 pounds, squatting over 500 pounds and running below a 4.7 in the 40-yard dash. In all honesty, I was convinced that that was all I needed to do. I had this idea that improving my strength, speed and simply working hard at practice and games, would have me on my way. After enduring my foot injury and losing my power, speed, agility and explosiveness, I was humbled and willing more than ever to try anything and everything that would help me to regain my prior athletic abilities.

One of the most common questions I'm asked, is regarding the one most important component of this method. We have a tendency to want to be bottom-lined. The simple answer is: *all of it*. Each component is beneficial for each athlete. One part will be more useful to some athletes over others, and that's because every athlete has his or her own set of weaknesses that need to be attended to. There is no way to tell, without a proper evaluation, what the most critical thing is for an athlete to work on, in any given moment.

If you coach at the college or professional level, this method will not only make your team more competitive--improving the athletic performance of the athletes you have--but it will keep your athletes healthier, at a higher rate. This is equally true for coaches of high school athletics--but hopefully, with less stress involved, and fewer jobs on the line.

If I had come across this early in my career, it would have saved me an exceptional amount of time and money. I have read countless books, have attended several different seminars, and spent hours testing out what I was learning, to see if it worked or not. Most of what I had learned or read, simply did not work when I put it to the test of training hard. Many things made me feel better, and in fact improved my range of motion or some other area of my athleticism--however, it did not stick. The only things which have worked for both my athletes and myself, can be found here in this book.

The part which can be difficult to accept, is that despite me sharing with you exactly what we do in order to help our athletes perform at their best, it still takes skill to make sure it all works. Let's take a world famous chef and an average cook, as an example. Yes, the famous chef can write down step by step cooking instructions for the cook to follow--but in the end, the food likely doesn't taste the same. What happens, is that there are always moving parts because of temperature, and quality of ingredients. This is something that a seasoned chef can work around, because of the depth of experience that they have accumulated throughout their career. An average cook, is limited to just the book and left to follow the steps--despite what may be less than ideal conditions. Something will naturally arise, which calls for a draw on experience to be properly dealt with. All this to say don't be too hard on yourself. Always continue to improve, because when you do that, you will get to a point where things will begin clicking, and you will have the experience to execute this method under any circumstance.

You will not regret the time you put into mastering this method, because not only will your athletes perform better, but you will be helping to decrease your team's overall injury rate by ninety five percent! Imagine working for a professional or college team which has just had a difficult season, due to injuries. You're left wondering what could have been done, or what can you do to help your team to not walk through the same hardships as last season. I myself, experienced that as a college athlete. Not only did I get hurt, but almost half of the starters were injured during that season--resulting in a singular win for the season, and our coaching staff ultimately being fired.

When I see teams and athletes that are facing constant injury, I tend to also see everyone chalking it up to bad luck. At one point, I may have agreed; but after putting in the research and testing, I've come to determine that this line of thinking is not only incorrect, but destructive. It's essentially removing the search for an answer, and leaving your fate in the hands of chance. I truly believe that some occasions of injury are unlucky. That being said, the majority of injuries are often 100% preventable. Does your coaching staff know how to prepare athletes in the proper way?

I've been an athlete my entire life. There is nothing that can make you care or know how important the small things are, until you go through such a huge failure like I experienced. It's due to those failures, that I continually push myself to find out why or how we can do it better. Without the emotional attachment that comes along with experiencing something of that nature, it's unlikely that one will put in the work to test things out, challenge preconceived notions, and not put anyone or a training method in higher regard than others. That is, unless they produce the desired results, time and time again.

In this book, I try to make it as easy as possible for you to grasp what we do, and how we do it. I've had several different business coaches advise me to franchise the business, because we deliver something so unique. Education, however, is what's at our heart. We know that majority of athletes who come to us, are clueless about what to focus on, and the order in which things should be done. I am a firm believer in the words of one of my great coaches, "...We can give them our play book and they can know exactly what we are running, but if we play with heart and execute 100%, it will not matter." Please read this and go out and execute this 100%, because the people you are helping need all of it.

THE
DM
ATHLETICS
TRAINING
METHOD

Step 1: Nutrition Evaluation

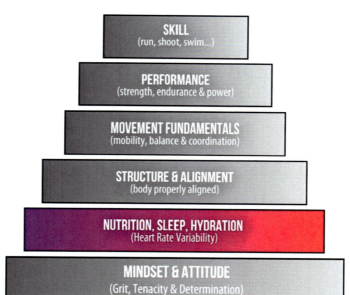

The first step in our training method, always involves assessing an athlete's nutrition. We begin by measuring their vitamin and mineral levels, because good nutrition is key in keep them healthy, long-term. Their food and liquid intake, along with sleep and proper breathing, are all vital to the training process. Unfortunately, most athletes do not take in enough food to perform their best, nor do they eat the right kinds of food or drink enough water. If an athlete's nutrition is not professionally analyzed and monitored, it's impossible to know whether they are getting all of the necessary vitamins, minerals, and calories. When athletes sign up to work with us, we immediately have them schedule a nutrition assessment with our naturopath. The earlier that an athlete's nutrition is assessed and adjusted, the faster they will begin to achieve results.

When the athlete's vitamin and mineral levels are extremely low in any area, the body begins to take what it needs from the bones, ligaments, or muscles, resulting in a higher chance of injury. Furthermore, their energy level, recovery, and performance will be compromised under such conditions. There's no end to the number of nutritional supplement companies, which claim to target this problem. They market their products to athletes, coming off as a seemingly one-size-fits all approach, which will guarantee success. While there are in fact some great products on the market, without a proper nutrition analysis, it's impossible to know exactly which supplement (and what form of that supplement) is appropriate. We strive for accuracy in all aspects of improving athletic performance--including nutrition--so this is not something we're comfortable leaving up to chance. We don't want to guess which foods and supplements will enhance performance. Instead, with the help of nutritionists, we create individualized nutritional plans for each of our athletes, based on the data gathered from the assessment of their blood work.

According to the *American College of Sports Medicine,* in order to provide the best nutritional support for an athlete, their nutritional recommendations need to be individualized because every athlete has a different height, weight, and body type. Varying demands from their sport and their training program, also play into determining what their bodies need to perform at its best. This means that any cookie cutter approach used by nutrition and supplement companies, cannot possibly be the best suited for each individual athlete. Yes, they may cover the basics. But to see the best results, you need to get a detailed review of what you need and how to implement it into your everyday food intake.

The College also recommends that athletes should not follow nutritional plans that deplete the energy levels and cognitive function during training and competition. There is a big movement out there to avoid carbohydrates. It may work well for some workout programs, but for an athlete that competes, carbohydrates are extremely important for supplying the energy they need--especially toward the end of competitions, when you need to dig deep and give it everything you've got.

We had a professional fighter who followed a no carbohydrate meal plan, despite our strong recommendation not to. He exclaimed how he felt great, and wouldn't want to give that up, just prior to his big fight. He felt great in training, and was confident that he would do well in his fight. Along came the day of the fight, and he was in fact still performing well. He felt great after the first round, but in the middle of the second round, things took a turn for the worse. His energy level was down and we could see it. He could not move as quickly as he did when the fight had begun, and spent the last two rounds just trying to stay in it. He lost that fight and after evaluating everything he did leading up to the fight, he realized that his diet was the only thing he had changed in his preparation--this time, resulting in the only instance in which he felt like he had completely lost his energy during a fight. Since he's made the change back to a more diet with incorporates some amount of carbohydrates, he has not lost a fight, since. We are hoping that Demetrious "Mighty Mouse" Johnson continues to win all of his fights until he retires.

The main goal of an athlete's nutritional plan is to provide nutritional support; allowing the athlete to perform their best, recover, and remain injury free during practice, training and competition. There is a direct link between not having the proper nutritional support and injury. Don't take a chance on a nutritional plan that you've received from a friend or someone that is not a professional. Your health is relying on it! Get with the right people, who will take the necessary steps to make sure you're at your best.

In addition to eating the proper foods, it's vital that you are drinking the right amount of water to stay properly hydrated throughout the day. The vast majority of people do not drink enough water, and experience the signs of dehydration without even realizing it. Headaches, low energy, feelings of hunger, dry skin, and dry lips, can all be signs of dehydration. This next part varies, but the recommended amount of water we should drink is 8 to 12 glasses a day. That is anywhere from 64 to 96 ounces of water, for the atypical person. For athletes, that number is higher, as you need more water to replace the amount of liquids you lose during workouts, practice and games.

A safe estimate would be to drink half of your body weight, in ounces of water each day. Now, we're just talking water. You can of course drink additional sports drinks or juice for electrolytes--but water is truly the most important component to staying hydrated. When you are dehydrated for a workout, practice or game, your performance will suffer dramatically.

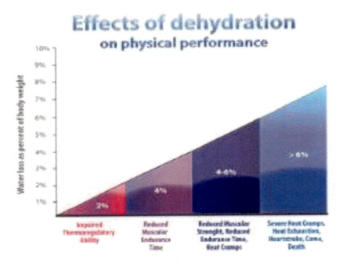

As you can see demonstrated in this graph, losing just 2% of your water weight will trigger the start of a decline in performance. The more water you lose without replacing it, the greater the risk of muscle cramps, reduced muscle strength, and even heat stroke, coma and death. Sure, coma and death seem extreme-- but in some cases, athletes have pushed themselves to the extreme. We are trained to push past the pain and to continue working hard no matter what is going on in our bodies. As a result, we often turn off our natural response to signs of danger.

Sometimes heat is the cause of dehydration, and that's one factor that we don't have control over. I can recall watching a game where the temperature was over 90 degrees, and the athletes on the field were cramping up. They had to stop playing more than ten times, to help an athlete off the field due to cramps. I was astonished because I had never witnessed it at that frequency before. I recall wondering why the game couldn't be postponed until night, when the temperature would drop. In those types of cases, you need to insist that athletes are drinking something.

Another reason why athletes tend to dehydrate, is because many people just do not like to drink anything while they're in competition. It may sound counterproductive, but the athlete's focus is so centered around the competition, that they forget the basic need to drink water or any other form of liquid. Some athletes forget to take a breath during competition, and that too, poses other problems. I am sure we can all relate to a time when we were so focused on what we were doing, that we forgot to eat or even to do other basic things. As coaches and parents, we need to constantly remind our athletes to drink water during competition.

There is some evidence out there, suggesting that pickle juice can stop cramping faster than water. Drinking it prior to physical activity, may even help prevent cramping. Pickle juice contains twenty times the amount of sodium, and eight times the potassium as the leading sports drinks. You only need one to two ounces of it; according to Kevin Miller and colleagues at North Dakota State University and Brigham Young University. Their studies have shown that it is more effective than marketed beverages, alleviating cramps in an average of thirty seconds.

One of our clients--an NFL athlete--suffered a constant stream of injuries. Two were major, and there were several additional minor injuries. When we analyzed his nutrition, we found that he had many vitamin and mineral deficiencies. He began taking the proper supplements to normalize his levels, while simultaneously making the necessary dietary adjustments to ensure that he would eventually get those vitamins and minerals from food based sources. Within a month, he had more energy, was recovering better, and slept better. His performance improved accordingly, and in his thirteenth season in the NFL, he made the Pro Bowl for the first time in his career. There were a number of elements to his training program that contributed to enhanced performance, but the nutritional adjustments were a foundational component of his results.

Let's use a personal example of how nutrition affects performance and recovery. When I was in High School, I made a goal of benching 500 pounds. At the point at which I was lifting 425 pounds relatively easily, I ended up getting hurt and was unable to regain my strength. In College, I saw some improvement on that goal, but then the same thing ended up happening. Whenever I approached benching 500 pounds, I would get hurt. This led me to eventually have my vitamin and mineral levels analyzed. To my shock, I discovered that I was deficient in a variety of different vitamins. I immediately changed my diet, and began supplementing appropriately. The difference I felt, happened pretty quickly. After the changes, it took just two months for me to finally bench 500 pounds.

I worked for more than fifteen years, to accomplish a goal I had set in High School. Though I had experimented with different training programs and philosophies, it wasn't until after I finally addressed nutrition, that I was able to understand my issues with meeting my goal. Some people may assert that I'm crazy for working on the same goal for so long; but I knew that I was capable of accomplishing it. Athletes should always continue pressing, until they achieve their goals. Sometimes they will fail along the way, but failure can serve us. Failure shows us that it's necessary to try another path or a new technique. It may be hard to see in the moment, but upon reflection, it becomes clear as to how important each failure was, on the path to growth and success.

Identify a Naturopath or another health care provider, that can work with you to run nutritional blood tests on your athletes. Many coaches are not taking this step, and some athletes will want to skip over it. In the event that they are resistant, do not allow them to skip this step.

Step 2: Posture Evaluation.

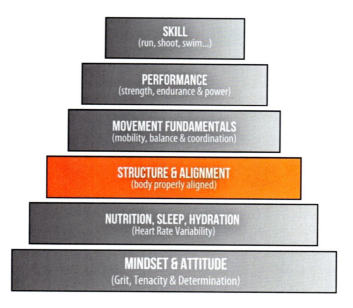

Once a nutritional assessment has been conducted, we move on to photographing the athlete's posture, in order to determine his or her weaknesses. This step makes our facility unique. Many training facilities skip it, because it's unpopular or is viewed as being outside the scope of athletic training. However, we view addressing posture as a critical step. There's a common misperception that posture can be corrected by simply standing a certain way--but it's much more involved than that. The problems which surface, are due to daily activities that hold our bodies out of alignment. Activities such as sitting for long durations of time, driving, walking in a particular way, injuries, accidents and so forth. They each contribute to our bodies falling out of alignment. Our goal with the modalities we utilize, is to bring the body slowly back into alignment and keep it there. We've worked with several different philosophies, but prefer the one we utilize, best, as it can be given to our athletes as part of their warm up.

I was introduced to this training element after suffering from a knee injury that wouldn't heal. I spent two and a half years visiting every health care provider I could find, to help me overcome my knee pain. Everything I tried, did in fact help to a certain degree; however, the pain was never 100% gone. Each professional that I consulted, advised me to stop lifting weights and playing basketball, because of the pain. I loved playing basketball and weightlifting, so I was reluctant to agree to giving those activities up. I had to continue looking for solutions and trying new things, until I was able to eliminate the pain.

During my quest to eliminate my knee pain, I read a book titled *Pain Free* by Pete Egoscue. It discussed the important role that posture plays in eliminating pain. I met with a posture therapist who photographed my posture, and it became clear from the photos, that my posture was the root cause of my knee pain. For three solid months, I threw myself into the program which the therapist recommended. This helped to correct my posture, which resulted in my knee pain disappearing during lifting and basketball, for the first time in years. In addition, my lifts actually improved alongside my posture. Here I was in my thirties, finally achieving some of the fitness goals that I had been working on since high school. This is what led to convincing me to including posture evaluation in our training method.

The further I looked into it, the more surprised I became by the fact that the method had been around for so long, but never talked about in any training material, articles or research that I had come upon. The founders have worked with several professional athletes--even Hall of Famers in the NFL--who utilized the method to stay healthy during their careers. This was a turning moment for me, as it was the point at which it became clear to me, that everything which was getting attention on the subject, was looking at the problem from one perspective. After realizing this, I knew I would never find the answer to what I was seeking, if I continued searching in the same places. I needed to broaden my scope to include topics which rarely were discussed. Topics which almost seemed unrelated to strength training and recovery. We all have blind spots, and it's human nature for a group of people in the same field to lose sight of what the answer could be, because everyone is looking at it from the same angle. This is why it is so important to include different kinds of people on your team--or at the very least, expose yourself to several different perspectives. We each hold a different view of the same problem. Only recently, did I learn that one of the guys I've long admired in the training realm, is learning and appreciating the Egoscue Method. To know that others in the industry are now catching on, is exciting.

After photographing the athlete's posture, we review the images with them, in order to develop a mutual understanding of the problem(s). The majority of people have no idea that their posture is an issue, but it becomes clear to them upon being presented with the photos.

Next, we conduct a postural evaluation to learn the range of motion for the athlete's hips and shoulders. This evaluation is used to confirm what is demonstrated by the photos. Athletes are able to feel their restrictions during this evaluation because of their weaknesses. This allows us to determine a range-of-motion baseline for where they started; having this baseline allows us to document improvement over time.

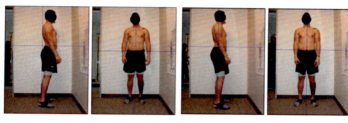

Before					After

The photos above, illustrate what we are trying to accomplish. The two photographs on the left were taken as part of an assessment, prior to instituting any corrective training program. The two photographs on the right, which were taken after the athlete completed his training program, show that his alignment has significantly improved. The ear, shoulder, hip and ankle are more aligned. The pelvic tilt and the head position has also improved.

This is when the buy in from our athletes take place. When they see that their posture is not in alignment, it is hard to debate. We can tell them what's wrong with them and they might even agree but when they see it and have a clear visual for us to explain the issues that we need to fix, there is no argument.

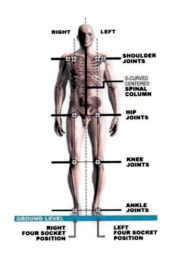
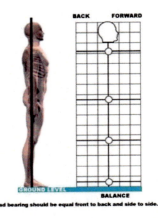

Load bearing should be equal front to back and side to side.

We compare our athlete's picture to what an aligned body looks like. They often ask, "is anyone properly aligned?" The answer is no. People that live in countries where they sit all the way down to their ankles to rest and stay active all day, have a greater chance of being in alignment. Where people sit in chairs or drive cars, their bodies will adapt to the lifestyle of doing those things. We as a species, were never designed to sit all day or be in cars or planes, for hours on end. Doing these things has an effect on the body and it has to adapt. While we can't change the fact that people have to sit down in chairs or drive in cars all day, we can give them a set of exercises that will help their bodies come back into alignment.

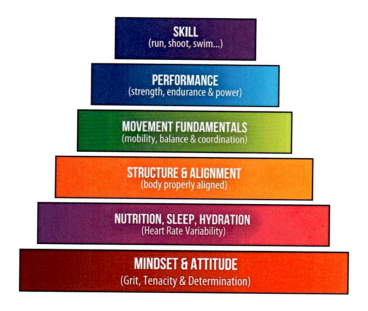

Here is the performance pyramid which illustrates the importance of each component that we focus on. The structure and alignment of the body is the foundation of the training portion of the pyramid. When you neglect this, you fail to give your athletes the strongest foundation to build their athleticism upon. Most coaches go straight to working on strength, power, explosiveness and endurance; but if they have poor alignment and movement fundamentals, injuries will occur. The body will overcompensate for any weakness or misalignment in it. Increased attention needs to be placed on the alignment, as it will inevitably improve everything else you focus on. Whether it be movement, strength, power, explosiveness or even skill set--these are all affected by alignment.

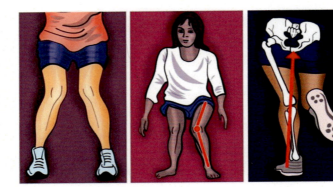

Above, is an example of knee valgus. Knee valgus s is the greatest indicator of future knee injuries. Using the Egoscue Method, we are able to correct this in our athletes. When the knee and hips are in this alignment, it places great pressure on the knee-- leading to a non-contact ACL or MCL injury. This is more common amongst women, because of how the hips are structured in relation to their knees. It can be fixed, so don't feel as though you're destined to inevitable problems. It is important however, to be alert to the fact that female athletes need more attention in this area.

One of our athletes, a football player at Harvard University, had experienced knee pain for years. He worked with several physical therapists and doctors to alleviate the pain, in order to play without issue. Despite playing for one of the leading college institutions in the country, he was unable to obtain effective help for his pain. When we began working with him, we photographed his posture and he followed the program which we had created for him. After just six weeks of working with us, he was able to play football again, without any knee pain. He was so excited to be able to engage in his favorite activities again--pain-free. This was a rewarding moment not only for him, but also for everyone who had helped him through the process. It was one of those moments where we were reminded why we started in this industry.

Postural Restoration Institute

There is another method which we like to utilize, to get our athletes get back into alignment. The Postural Restoration Institute (PRI) utilizes breathing, while positioning the body in various ways, to get all areas back into alignment. Their evaluation system determines what the athlete needs to work on first--and progressing until they've returned to alignment, and are moving better.

The exercises take just ten to fifteen minutes to complete; making them perfect to give to our athletes prior to their workout. Do we utilize the use of Physical Therapists? Absolutely. Their skill level is so particular, that when an issue is beyond our scope of knowledge, we refer them to the therapist we trust.

The key with these exercises, is that the results are quick, and athletes can feel an immediate difference.

I point out these various methods, because I want to highlight the fact that there are options which can be used--even at times, alongside each other. Don't get stuck or set on one. Both of these methods have been useful for us, and we utilize pieces of each in training our athletes daily.

Similar to the first step, find an alignment therapist that you can refer your athletes to. The thing I look for is something my athletes can do for fifteen minutes or less before a workout, practice or game. If it takes too long, they usually won't do it. Building these relationships are important both for helping your athletes, but also for gaining deeper insight into alignment and performance related knowledge. Although we've taken the time to attain certification in these two forms of structural work, we don't hesitate calling on more experienced eyes to review our athletes. Knowing the terms which structural therapists use, gives us a means of speaking to our athletes about the topic. It's always important to be able to explain why you're doing what you're doing.

Step 3: Mobility Screening.

DM ATHLETICS TRAINING PYRAMID

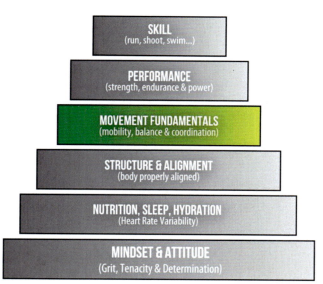

After assessing athletes' postures, conducting a functional movement test and determining athletes' weaknesses, we use a movement screen to critique how they move. The same weaknesses which were identified in the previous step, tend to also present themselves in this test--allowing us to explain to athletes how these restrictions limit their performance. We usually see that the hips or back are tight, and when we are able to loosen them, the athlete is able to take his or her performance to the next level.

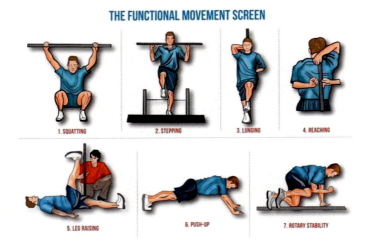

The following movements are performed as part of the screen:

1. The Deep Squat: tests mobility in the hips, lower back, and ankles.

2. The Hurdle Step: tests whether there is any restriction in the running motion.
3. The In-Line Lunge: measures whether there any restrictions when performing a lunge.
4. The Reaching test: determines whether the shoulders move properly.
5. The Active Straight Leg Raising (ASLR) test: checks hamstring flexibility and core stability.
6. The Trunk Stability Push-Up (TSPU) test: checks core and upper body strength.
7. The Rotary Stability test: checks shoulder and hip stability, when they work together.

Although ankle mobility is not examined by this screen, we consider it a vital element of athletic performance. The rest of the body (particularly knees and hips) must compensate, if there is an issue with the ankles. Therefore, we have created our own method of ensuring that our athletes retain good mobility in their ankles. We ask our athletes to sit on a bench, with one leg on the bench, and the ankle slightly off. Then we ask them to relax their foot and let it just hang; then bring it as far back toward their knee as possible. We utilize a tool which then measures the range of motion in degrees. Once that information is collected from both sides, we can see if it is normal or restricted. In most cases, people need to work on this. A cause may be the shoes we are wearing all day--restricting full range of motion in our ankles. It could also simply be the fact that we are sedentary the majority of the day. Whatever the case may be, this needs to have ten to twelve degrees of range of motion. If not, the hips and knees will overcompensate.

The theory behind testing and improving movement is that by doing so, it will improve performance. Imagine being restricted in certain movements when you are in competition. If we can open you up so those movements are no longer restricted, your performance will improve.

Jeff Fish, the strength and conditioning coach for the Phoenix Suns, promotes the functional movement test along with several other experts in the collegiate and professional strength coaching world. They have seen a drop in injuries and have been able to help their athletes perform at their best utilizing these test.

One of the things that Jeff realized when administering this test at the NFL combine for seven years, is that the average score of the athletes had not changed at all. They are focusing so much on getting bigger, faster and stronger, that they are negating the fundamental part of their training--which helps to explain why injuries continue to increase in the NFL (and throughout other sports as well). It's exciting to work on things which have a direct impact on your performance--whether it be speed, explosiveness or power. It's not difficult to see why the imbalance occurs.

The problem with this, is that when you continue to work on these things and pay little to no attention to things that need your attention (movement, structure) it is only a matter of time before your foundation ends up being tested. The injury rate if you make it to the NFL is 100%. If you play football in high school, then college, and are lucky enough to make it to the NFL, the chances of you getting hurt is 100%. Now, the degree of injury you endure will be dependent mainly on your structure, movement and the circumstances you find yourself in on the field. There are so many things which happen on the field that you just cannot control. The components that you can take care of, should be taken into account in an athlete's training program.

Athletes sometimes have a problem with changing direction, despite being incredibly fast. When their movement pattern is fixed, their ability to change direction naturally, improves without having to work on technique. One of our best examples of this, was a high school linebacker who started at 4.6 seconds in the pro agility shuttle. He dropped to 3.8 seconds, over the course of six months of training. He then went on to have the best season of his high school career, and was named defensive MVP for his conference. This led to being offered a full scholarship to play in college. We didn't even work on his technique, but instead on his structure and movement which was limiting his ability to accelerate, decelerate and change direction. The problem with working on technique, is that it pays no attention to what is going on in the athlete's body. By forcing a body which is experiencing ground floor issues, into a position that it is uncomfortable, you are only create larger problems. Also, when the athlete gets back on the field, they will inevitably return to what is most comfortable for their body to do. All of the time spent on working on technique, will not be utilized during competition if the other components have been left unaddressed.

If there is something that I wish I had been introduced to during my football career, it would have been the movement screen. Unfortunately, I wasn't introduced to the functional movement screen until I had an NFL tryout. I performed so horribly during the screen, that in hindsight, my tryout was practically over before it even started. The screen identified so many things to work on that had never come across my path. I had trained for the vertical jump, board jump, bench press, 40-yard dash, pro agility, and three-cone drill. When I was training, I didn't pay attention to my movement patterns because I didn't know how to work on them—in fact, I didn't even know that I *should* work on them. Instead, I focused on lifting weights, which was a strength of mine and something I enjoyed. As a result, my performance on the field deteriorated as my movement declined, following my foot injury.

I point this out, because this is why it's critical to focus on an athlete's weaknesses rather than continuing to focus on their strengths. Most athletes have an area of strength, but only a rare few have it all (strength, explosiveness, movement and alignment). When we work with athletes, our goal is to help them develop in all of the areas, to become better athletes. Strength and explosiveness can be improved, to a certain degree. Helping athletes improve alignment and movement will take their athleticism to another level.

Step 4: Performance and Growth Tracking.

DM ATHLETICS TRAINING PYRAMID

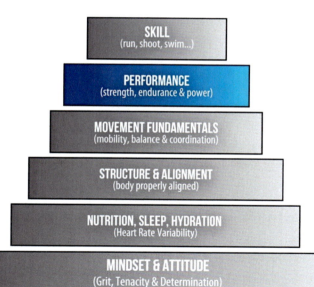

After assessing movement, we measure the athlete's vertical jump, strength, speed, and agility to determine a baseline of current athletic ability. It's vital that everyone know exactly where they are, especially when beginning. We use the vertec to measure vertical jump, a stopwatch to measure the pro agility shuttle, and to measure their straight ahead speed, we measure the 10 yard sprint and 20 yard sprint. In some cases, we measure a 40 yard sprint, but we like to stick to the 10 and 20 as the risk of injury is really low.

The fact that many facilities do not complete this step, never fails to surprise me. Numerous athletes come to our facility after working with other coaches. When we discuss their goals, I always ask about their baseline data, yet they typically don't have any measurements. In other words, they don't know where they started from, so it's difficult to determine just how much they've improved. The sheer number of people who spend years working out without measuring their performance and growth, is shocking.

Many athletes and coaches assume that feeling and looking better equates to performing better, but this is not the case. The only way to determine athletic progress is through unbiased measurements. I've been told many times, that a particular athlete looks unbelievable but can't play well. This is the consequence of when athletes work hard, but fail to test and measure the right performance metrics to help them prepare for their sport. The result is that they look amazing when they train, yet do not perform well in practice and games.

A basketball athlete came to in after training at another facility for two years. His main objective was to improve his vertical jump, because he wanted to dunk. I asked for his current vertical measurement, and he was unable to answer. I asked when he last tested his vertical and he said he never tested his vertical before. I was surprised, because he cited improving his vertical as the reason he sought training at his former facility. We established a baseline of 26", and after five months of training with us and utilizing our method, he had a 36" vertical jump and can now easily dunk.

This step is pretty simple. Track what your athletes are doing. You want to be able to show them improvement. Without this information, it is easy for athletes-- especially the younger ones--to lose engagement and not give it their all. Progress energizes people, and gives them the confidence that they can do better. I cannot stress how important this step is to the process. Track, track and track!

In Dr. Sean Young's book, *Stick to It*, he emphasizes the importance of tracking and setting small, short term goals that people can achieve. Yes it is good to have a big goal in the back of your mind, but having something concrete that you can achieve in a week, will keep athletes more engaged and put in more effort.

You might set goals such as playing at the college or professional level. Those are not bad goals to have. The problem is that if that is the only focus, studies show that people will lose interest and not give the effort needed, to realize their potential. With these as the ultimate goal, we can formulate a plan for our athletes to increase their athleticism gradually until they reach the level of a collegiate athlete.

For example--let's say a kid comes to us with a goal of playing college football. His vertical is 20 inches, 40 yard dash is 5.6 seconds, pro agility is 5.2, and he is a freshman linebacker. We would identify the average collegiate football player at his position, and how he is performing in all those drills. Then we would plan a goal that he can reach in a week, a month, three months, and eventually where he should be by his Senior year.

By doing things this way, we focus on the most important things we need to be doing right now. Progressing from his starting numbers to those which will have him ready for college, will take time. Most people do not have the patience to see it through. However, when they begin making small improvements, they see themselves getting closer to their goal and it becomes more of a reality. Just taking these small steps, are incredibly beneficial.

It's also important to celebrate the small gains which are made. Most athletes make improvements and want to hurry up and keep going, in an effort to get to their ultimate goal. In a sense, we all have a tendency to do this, as we become so hyper-focused on end results. The problem with this is that we leave ourselves no time for reflection and celebration.

The research is clear. When we take time to reflect on our accomplishments and celebrate a little, we give ourselves the energy to continue. Our brain releases dopamine when we set a goal and achieve it. The positive feelings we get from the release of dopamine, is what continues to drive us to take the next step. That's all we want our athletes to focus on; the next step.

As coaches, we also like to let their parents and friends know about their progress. This enables community support for their efforts. We all need encouragement from our family and our friends, and it gives us confidence to not only continue, but to put in more effort. Parents and friends will normally congratulate the athlete, which in turn releases more dopamine into the body. The athlete naturally devotes themselves further into their training, and they begin viewing it as a part of their everyday life.

This is the point at which they've decided that their training is non-negotiable.

Sharing their progress happens in various ways. Sometimes it's through emailing and talking to the parents, but it can also be through posting on social media. We love recognizing our athletes for their accomplishments in the gym, and have several athletes that have gone on to perform well enough to garner some publicity. It's become part of normal protocol for us to look out for their articles, and post them to our social media pages. We always look forward to tagging our athletes, and congratulating them for a great job.

It is an honor for us to be a part of the process which helps our athletes to reach their highest level of performance--but it all links back to tracking. Because we track their progress, we're able to keep them focused on the everyday grind, and how that will help their performance measures. We then reflect and celebrate each and every victory. Next, we take the community approach, and increase the number of people who have a genuine interest in, and can congratulate and encourage the athlete by letting those people know of their successes. When the athlete is having an off day and doesn't feel like training (as we all do), they'll have more than a coach to answer to. There will be more people encouraging the athlete to continue and not give up. By creating this kind of environment, you increase your chances of getting athletes to stick to it until they achieve their ultimate goal, not giving up beforehand.

Dr. Jean Cote, a professor and Director in the School of Kinesiology and Health Studies at Queen's University, found that youth tend to rate "excitement/challenge of competition" as one of their top reasons for sports participation. In other words, youth play sports because it is fun and challenging. When asked why they drop out of sports, they rarely mention any factors associated with keeping score; however, they discuss reasons related to lack of fun and increased pressure. Tracking your athletes-- regardless of age--will not deter them from participating; instead, it has quite the opposite effect.

In *The 4 Disciplines of Execution: Achieving Your Wildly Important Goals* by Chris McChesney, Sean Covey, and Jim Huling; they note a story of a scoreboard which had been turned off, at a high school football game. Coaches noticed that their players were less engaged, subconsciously putting in less effort than they had, prior. The crowd followed the same pattern and lost interest, as they not only did not know the score, but were unaware of how important the play on the field was, in relation to the outcome of the game.

When you fail to track the results of your athletes, they not only eventually lose interest, but they miss out on the critical support which is vital to their performance.

Professional Athletes

When training professional athletes, the motivation changes. The first thing you have to determine is whether your athlete has a fixed or a growth mindset. In *Mindset,* Dr. Carol Dweck discusses how athletes fall into one of two categories. First, is the fixed mindset, where the assumption is that everything is based on talent, and there is there is little which can be achieved by working hard. This will be covered in greater depth in the final chapter. The growth mindset holds the belief that effort impacts outcome, significantly. It is those with a growth mindset, that you can have a huge impact on.

You may be able to impact the career of an athlete with a fixed mindset, but it is more difficult because you are dealing with beliefs which are deeply seated in their belief systems. To unravel this and change their mindset, requires quite a bit of work, and may not be something that's in your wheelhouse of operation, Nevertheless, I encourage you to try. High school and college students tend to be open to suggestions, and are very teachable. They can be taught that their effort plays integral role in their success.

An athlete that has reached the professional ranks with minimal effort as a result of being extremely physically blessed, will likely be less open to suggestions. Because they were able to make it as-is, they'll tend to feel that their success is completely based on talent. Consequently, they may not put as much work into their craft.

I have a friend who I used to train with, back in Hawai`i. He saw me pushing myself hard in the weight room one day, and stated, "Why are you working so hard? You've either got it or you don't." This guy was an NFL vet, who had played ten seasons in the NFL. He clearly didn't push himself that hard and yet was able to play at the highest level, for a decade. What he failed to note, was that he had been injured several times, and never had an outstanding career. He was in fact an NFL player--but had he put in the hard work, he likely would have played longer, made more money, and have been remembered by fans after his career. This wasn't the case.

I like to begin with goals. I ask athletes, "You are a professional athlete now--so what are your new goals?" If they respond that it's a contract year, the goal typically has to do with keeping themselves strong on the radar. Depending on their level of athleticism and their career, I ask, "Do you want to be a Hall of Fame player?" You have to know who you're talking to, to gauge whether they're even open to new levels. Most will say yes, though when you proceed with asking whether they've studied any Hall of Fame players, the answer is often no. This is when I discuss the mindset that most Hall of Fame players have, in addition to their work ethic on the field, and in the gym.

It's not surprising to come to the realization that many pro level athletes are just as athletic, or close to being as athletic, as some Hall of Fame players. The catch is that they need to work on specific areas of which they're falling short on. Each athlete is unique, and the intensity of the conversation will vary.

Once you get them to buy in, you can proceed to follow the above steps. Motivation changes once you reach the professional level, so your approach and coaching style needs to adjust as well. It's a small adjustment which is worth the work.

Tracking the progress of professional athletes is super critical in comparison to that of high school and college athletes. Results will not be as drastic, at this level. In high school and college, there is a lot of room for improvement. By the time an athlete has reached the professional level, they are fully developed. They tend to be fast, explosive and strong. The gains they achieve will be slow, but they will be steady, given you've got them on the right program.

To demonstrate the contrast, let's compare a high school athlete to a professional athlete. It's pretty common in our facility, to help a high school athlete improve their pro agility shuttle by half a second, improve their vertical by five or more inches and drop their 40 by at least three tenths of a second during the off season. With a professional athlete, the goal would be to drop their pro agility three tenths of a second. Perhaps increase their vertical by three inches, and drop a tent or two off of their 40. These are athletes which are already jumping 35 inches in their vertical, and are already considered fast. These small incremental improvements do in fact have a dramatic impact on their performance on the field. The slightest increase in speed and explosiveness will allow them to make more plays. The result of that, are better contracts and increased success in their career.

We had a high school basketball athlete see a 14 inch increase in their vertical, after an off season spent with us. That however, would never be the case with one of our professional players. One of our great successes with our pro athletes, in the same arena, was a seven inch improvement in his vertical. Although it was half the number of inches as the high school athlete, it had greater impact, as he was beginning at a higher level. Any small improvement you can help your athlete achieve will only add to his effectiveness on the court or the field.

Step 5: Personalized Programs.

DM ATHLETICS TRAINING PYRAMID

- **SKILL** (run, shoot, swim...)
- **PERFORMANCE** (strength, endurance & power)
- **MOVEMENT FUNDAMENTALS** (mobility, balance & coordination)
- **STRUCTURE & ALIGNMENT** (body properly aligned)
- **NUTRITION, SLEEP, HYDRATION** (Heart Rate Variability)
- **MINDSET & ATTITUDE** (Grit, Tenacity & Determination)

Once we've gathered the aforementioned information and establishing the athlete's goals, our staff works together to draw up a personalized program. The program typically targets the main areas of weakness, which were identified in the posture assessment and movement screen. Attack an athlete's weaknesses prior to sharpening their strengths, yields greater improvement across all areas of athletic performance. If they're experiencing a difficult time changing direction but display great explosiveness, for instance, addressing agility issues will make the athlete more competitive.

If an athlete is coming off of an injury and needs to perform with the absence of any injury related problems the following season, then this step is more critical than ever. Be sure that when you are working with someone who is coming off an injury, they've been cleared for training by a physical therapist prior to starting. It's not uncommon to find athletes who are coming off of injuries, yet participating in the same activities which all of the other athletes in their program are participating in. There is clearly something wrong with an athlete that has been injured. Having them participate in the same exact workout program as the others, is not the answer.

Depending on the athlete's age, the program might begin by focusing only on weight lifting or doing body weight exercises. At the junior high, high school, and sometimes even college level, we find that many want to begin training by first doing heavy lifting. Instead, we have to press pause until their alignment and movements indicate that they are ready for higher-level activity; like lifting weights (ie, squats, cleans, and snatches).

Using the same program to train every athlete regardless of an individual's sport, unique strengths and weaknesses, is one of the primary reasons that injuries continue to happen. Yes, it is ideal to eventually get all of the athletes on a single team to use the same program for the sake of simplicity and ease of instruction. However, when they first begin training, it's most effective to focus attention on the areas of greatest concern for each individual player, rather than trying to apply a generic program to the entire team.

We've worked with several teams, and I won't pretend that it isn't difficult to accomplish. But I promise you, that the rewards you get from doing this, will far exceed the time spent developing each individual athletes' specific correctives or structural exercises. Besides, after you run the structural and movement screens, it will tell you what each athlete needs to do, to improve his or her weakness. I don't want coaches to get overwhelmed by having a couple of little different things for each person, but rather looking at it from the perspective of sprinkling in something small into the program, for each individual athlete. When you see it that way, it really doesn't seem so daunting. If you are coaching collegiate or pro athletes, this shouldn't be of concern, because this is precisely your job. For those that coach in a high school, or perhaps at the volunteer level, it can prove more difficult, as they often have a limited amount of time to do anything extra, beyond facilitating the workout.

I understand both sides of the spectrum, as I volunteered quite a bit, during the early days of my career. It's difficult to balance your full time job, coaching and family. Thankfully, I loved this stuff so much, that it was no problem for me to stay up late or wake up early, to continually work on refining my skill. For those who are short on the time it takes, to go through and individualize programs for their athletes, we can do it for you. By utilizing the results from the screens you have conducted and the program you have in mind, we are able to blend the two, and craft a program which will ensure that your athletes are getting exactly what they need, when they need it. Just contact us via our email, which can be found at www.dmathletics.com.

Our programs cater to each athlete's individual needs. For example, if an athlete begins with poor ankle mobility, we will first give them some exercises to address that particular problem, prior to moving on to other areas. At the same time, another athlete might have poor core strength and flexibility. That athlete's set of exercises would be completely different than that of the one with the ankle issues. This is really the only approach which makes sense; ankle exercises don't help to strengthen the core, and core exercises can't improve ankle mobility. This is why our individualized program is so critical to success.

When our high school athletes leave for college, they return weaker and slower than they were prior to leaving us. Most colleges insist that everyone on a team participate in the same training program; it's very unusual to find individual programs which cater to each athlete's specific needs. This happens because there are so many people on the team, and there are limited numbers of coaches available to work with them. There are 80 to 100 players on a college football team, for example, and the NCAA only allows five strength and conditioning coaches to work with all 80 to 100 of those athletes. With those ratios, it is difficult for anyone to get any individualized attention. It's difficult, but it can in fact, be done. Our college athletes make it a priority to come in as much as possible when they are home, because we can work with them individually or in a small group--ensuring that they get the attention they need to perform at their best.

There are a few exceptions, but college-level Head Strength Coaches who create individual programs for their athletes, are not the norm. They produce amazing results, but these results are often dismissed by other coaches who assume that the outstanding performance is due to natural athletic ability. That is, of course, true for the schools that get the top recruiting classes year in and year out. However, it is not the case for the schools whose recruits are in the middle of the pack, and are still able to compete or even beat the schools that regularly recruit the top players.

With the first couple of steps (posture and movement evaluation) it will reveal specific points that each individual athlete needs to work on. If you have a set program, just add it to parts of the program or make them do it before. In this way, everyone is doing the important things you want to get done but at the same time working on their own individual weakness. Only in this way will you be able to get the most out of your athletes, help them perform at their highest level and reduce the risk of injuries significantly.

In helping to avoid non-contact injuries during the season, you need to add single leg exercises into your programs. Incorporating single leg exercises, works muscles which are different that those you'd work by doing exercises with both feet on the ground. The groin, glute mead and balance, receive more focus than if you were to focus only on normal squats, deadlifts and cleans. There are several single leg exercises you can incorporate, and I recommend you implement as many as you can. You don't need to cover it all at once. It's most beneficial to start with easy single leg exercises, and then progress to more difficult ones when your athletes are ready.

All that being said, I don't advocate doing only single leg exercises, while avoiding heavy squats, deadlifts or cleans. I love all of those lifts, and believe they are extremely useful; but like anything else, too much of a good thing is simply too much. During any athletic competition, athletes utilize both coming off of two feet, and at other times one foot; so you need to train for both scenarios. While playing defensive line in college, and executing short yardage or goal line plays, we were expected to explode into our opponents off of two feet--getting as far into the back field, as possible. With this in mind, it's difficult to understand why some coaches in the industry do not advocate for incorporating heavy squats. When you're an athlete facing two three hundred pound guys who plan to dump you on your back, you will need all the power and mental toughness you can muster, to survive and win.

Here are the single leg exercises that we like to use with our athletes. The first ones are easiest, only to progress to more difficult ones, as she/he becomes ready. Once an athlete can get to the point at which they can do a single leg squat off a box (to parallel or lower), they reduce their risk of ACL injury by 90%.

1. Single Leg Squat with TRX

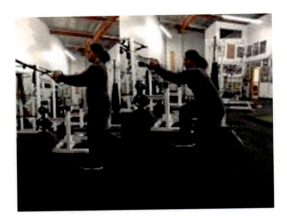

As you can see here, you want to get down as low as possible, using as little help from your hands. The goal is to eventually touch the knee to the ground.

2. Pistol Squats

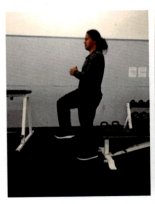 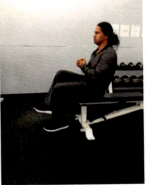

Pistols are great for strengthening the glutes, groin and balance. The key here is to control the whole motion. Do not just drop down. When you hit the bench, try and just tap it and then lift back up.

When I first tried this, I couldn't do it. I had just completed my college football career, and women in the gym were accomplishing this easily. That pushed me to work on it while I was alone--eventually getting to a point where I could add weight. Remember--if you haven't been doing single leg exercises, it will be difficult at the start. Just continue, and it will get easier. These help to improve your squats and deadlifts, because you're working muscles when doing the single leg exercises, which you don't when sticking solely to two legged exercises.

3. Hip Ups

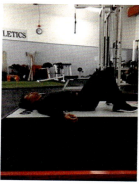
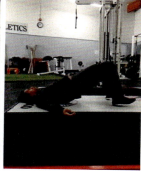

Hip ups are great for getting the glutes fired up and ready to go. Be sure that the line from your knee to your shoulder, is straight. If it's not straight when when you first begin, it's not a problem-- just keep working it until you get there.

When you reach the point at which you have everything lined up and it feels easier, add weight. Slowly add weight. The most important thing, is that you are executing it correctly.

4. Single Leg Hip Ups

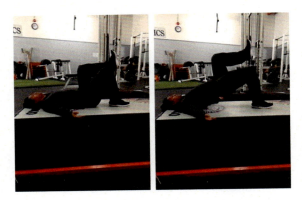

Similar to hip ups, but using just one leg, you'll continue trying to achieve a straight line from your hip to your shoulder. This is much more difficult to accomplish with one leg. When you are able to reach a point where everything is in alignment; add weight.

5. Rear Foot Elevated (RFE)

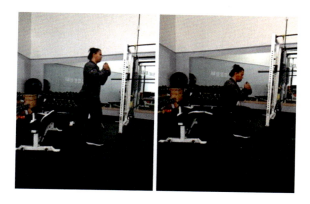

With this exercise, you can start with body weight then progress to adding weight. You can use a kettlebell, dumbbells in your hands, or a bar on your back. I love this exercise because not only are you working the leg with the foot on the ground, but you are also stretching the back leg.

I couldn't touch the ground with my knee when I first did this. Attempting to force it, didn't work either. However, as I continually pursued the exercise, it dropped slowly-- eventually to the point that it was meeting the ground. Don't force it--go to where your body allows you to go.

6. Slide Board Single Leg Squat

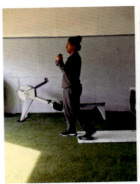 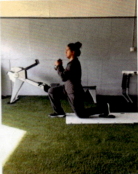

Similar to RFE, but with the utilization of the slide board. When the back leg is on the slide board, your hamstrings will be used more to get your body back up. Once again, begin without weight. Use only your body weight, until you can touch the back knee to the ground. Once you can lift yourself up easily, you can then feel free to add weight.

You can use a kettlebell, dumbbells in each hand or a bar on your back. I like to mix it up, as each one taxes your body in a different way.

7. Single Leg Squat Off Box

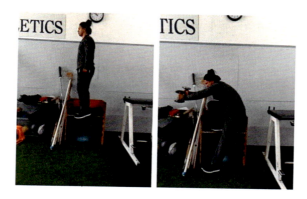

This is the granddaddy of them all. The goal here, is to get the athlete to be able to get to parallel level, or lower. You can start by lowering the box so that their foot hits the ground once they're parallel. Once they've achieved that, raise the box so that they cannot hit the ground.

The weights in the hand, aren't the most important detail. You only need 5 to 15lbs of weight. Obviously, the heavier the athlete, the more weight they will need to effectively counterbalance. Don't worry about adding crazy amounts of weight here. The goal is in the range of motion--as it is with all the other single leg exercises.

Like anything else, you don't want to become so focused on these exercises, that you neglect doing squats, deadlifts and cleans. They are all great exercises which should be done by all athletes. People tend to find something new, only to later abandon the old exercises which were working great. Remember--these are only to add to a program that already includes all of the staple leg exercises. It's not necessary to run through them all at once. Perhaps you can try two for a couple weeks, trading off for the other two, the following weeks. The primary goal is to get your athletes to be able to do the single leg squat off the box, to parallel or lower.

Step 6: Heart Rate Variability Monitoring.

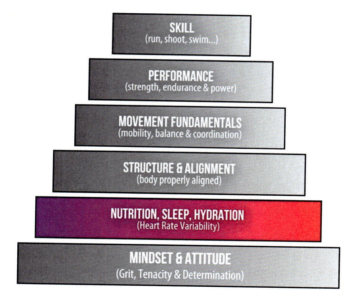

Once the training program is in place, we hook all of our pro athletes up to a Heart Rate Variability (HRV) system, which monitors their daily recovery during the training program. The athlete begins wearing a heart rate monitor at all times--monitoring sleep quality, exercise and HRV, daily. The reading will generate information which tells us whether or not the athlete is ready to train, take it easy that day, or take the day off.

We find this key to learning how our athletes are recovering. The data alerts coaches of any need to alter the training program, when athletes do not properly recover. There are many variables in an athlete's life which we as coaches are unable to control: family, relationships, stress, and so forth. These are the kinds of factors which can prevent the athlete's body from properly recovering, and being ready to workout and compete. HRV monitoring allows coaches to see--in real time--whether athletes are ready to train, need a lighter training day than usual (for instance, avoiding heavy weights and significant conditioning), or would benefit from a recovery day. Recovery days typically align with program scheduling, but each athletes has a unique recovery rate, so monitoring is beneficial.

Some athletes may have abnormal dysfunctions—even those of which they are unaware of. They can dictate a recovery that is longer than that of others on their team. In multiple cases, where an athlete has passed away after working out with their team, an autopsy is performed, only to reveal that they had a rare disease of which they were unaware of. These cases are rare, but for coaches that oversee big teams, it's well worth it to keep each of your athletes safe, with the hope of never experiencing a situation where someone's life is at risk.

There are HRV devices which monitor sleep quality; and that information is vital for a coach to have. On the coaches end, you're able to see how much sleep your athletes are getting, when they went to sleep, what time they woke up, and how much of their sleep was quality sleep versus tossing and turning. Sleep is the best thing athletes can do to recover from workouts, practices and games. According to the American Academy of Pediatrics, sleeping at least eight hours a night will reduce the risk of injury by 68%. It also improves an athlete's reaction time by 32%.

A study performed by Mah CD, Mah KE, Kezirian EJ, and Dement WC, examined the effects of sleep extension on the athletic performance of collegiate basketball players in 2011. They found that when basketball players slept for 10 hours a night, their free throws improved by 9%, while their three point shot improved by 9.2%. Improve your athlete's performance, while simultaneously dropping the risk of injury by 68%, just by ensuring that they're sleeping 8 to 9.5 hours a night.

The School of Kinesiology at Simon Frasier University, conducted a study on the effectiveness of HRV monitoring, when it comes to concussion athletes. They had 147 hockey athletes sign up to be monitored and tested. Of those 147, fourteen of them sustained a concussion during the season. When continuing to monitor their HRV, they found that there was a definite decrease in their HRV in light workout, three days after they were concussed. They continued to monitor them, and found that most athletes did not return back to normal, until seven days after their concussion. Some athletes took a little longer. The HRV monitoring was used with the normal concussion protocols they still use to this day, but the HRV was able to indicate when the athlete had actually returned back to normal.

The whole body is interconnected as one system. When the brain, cardiovascular or any other system is damaged, the whole system is affected, causing the heart to adjust. The body will always provide increased resources to the parts of the body which are infected, bleeding and damaged. By tracking HRV, you begin to be able to detect where there is a short circuit. It gives you the opportunity to take the necessary steps in order to get your athlete the proper help.

A study examining elite runners (spearheaded by Daniel J Plews), shows that monitoring HRV has tremendous benefits. Predicting recovery times and setting weekly training regimen that will not impede their training, is just one of them. By monitoring an athlete's HRV, they are able to predict when they'll need a day off, or will hit a wall in their training.

You don't want to push athletes to the point to which they're risking their health. Monitoring HRV allows coaches to take the guesswork out of training their athletes. When coaches are able to utilize this, they avoid the possibility of overtraining them, and also the health problems which are a result of overtraining.

In recent news, a college strength coach has made headlines for pushing his players to the point at which they had to be hospitalized on two different occasions. I am a big proponent for training an athletes mental component--pushing them beyond their comfort zone. However, never would I advocate going so far as to needing an ambulance to come and assist multiple participants. That is overtraining. Those kinds of issues can be easily avoided when HRV is monitored. It would be clear to the coach, that the athletes were not taking it easy, but were pushing themselves to the limit. Thankfully in this situation, nobody died. One student however, did have to avoid physical activity for three months, following the incident.

I have been the coach on the other side of the fence, wondering if some guys are just quitting on me, and not giving the practice everything they had. While I do push and motivate, I also err on the side of caution, as there's no way I will risk a negative outcome.

While training a group of high school students, we embarked on five hill runs. The hill was about 200 yards long. It got competitive, and the kids continued going after the five hills they had completed. I let it go on, as I admired their competitiveness. The day was extremely hot--above 90 degrees--so I announced that I didn't want them running more than eight hills, total. When they got to ten, I told them to stop and they refused. I then told the rest of the kids to head back to the weight room with me. When they reached hill sprint number fifteen, one of the kids passed out. When I was notified, I called 911 and had the kid rushed to the hospital. It was the scariest moment of my life as a coach because I was completely responsible for the situation. The kids didn't listen to me, but I could have grabbed each kid and forced them to stop. If I had an HRV monitoring system available to me, I could have forecasted the situation ahead for them, but at this point in my career, I did not. Thankfully the student recovered fully, after a night in the hospital--but it was a great lesson for me to learn. Force your athletes to stop when they are supposed to do so. The risk does not outweigh the reward, in situations such as these.

The Proper Way to Breathe

We are continuously looking for ways that our athletes will be able to maintain a competitive edge when they compete. It's amazing to me, how much the small details matter in performance. For years, I didn't realize that there's a proper way to breathe, in order to recover faster and perform at a higher level. Breathing is something we do without thinking, and thus it is something so small that the majority of us never consider if we're breathing in the most optimal way to perform our best. Breathing properly, positively influences our Heart Rate Variability (HRV). The more efficiently our athletes are able to get oxygen throughout their bodies during and after competition, the more of an advantage they will have

In his book, *The Oxygen Advantage,* Patrick McKeown demonstrates how mouth breathing is detrimental to sports performance and overall health. When you breathe through your mouth, a limited amount of oxygen reaches the diaphragm-- which is able to get oxygen to your organs faster. Breathing through your nose, allows your body to filter environmental toxins, while also adjusting temperature prior to reaching your diaphragm. Mouth breathing simply does not allow for these steps to take place. In addition, breathing through your mouth aids in the drying out of your mouth-- giving you an increased chance of dental problems.

How do we take this information and improve our sports performance? First, McKeown recommends that we begin breathing through our nose. If our mouth is dry upon waking, we can tape our lips while we sleep, to force ourselves to breathe through our nose. If you struggle with sleep apnea, this is not an avenue you want to pursue, as you need to breathe through your mouth at certain points in the night. Athletes can also breathe through their nose while recovering. During intense competition, they should be allowed to breathe however they breathe--but as soon as they are able, they should be encouraged to breathe through their nose between plays.

Athletes can also practice breath holding exercises, to improve how the body handles performing with a lack of oxygen. Take a normal breath through the nose, followed by a normal exhale. Immediately pinch your nose, and take as many steps as possible, inhaling as soon as you feel the first sign that you need to breathe. The goal is to reach a point where you can take 80 steps. Don't worry if you have a difficult time taking several steps. I'm in that group. Your ability to be more competitive at the end of games, will improve dramatically as the score goes up.

Eliminate Exercise Induced Asthma

Can you really eliminate exercise induced asthma? According to Patrick McKeown, it's 100%

preventable. When I learned this piece of information, it was eye opening. I had worked with several athletes who dealt with this condition. To find that there was a way to help them in this regard, got me excited. McKeown discusses athletic performance, and how breathing properly assists overall health. He further examines how proper breathing eliminates exercise induced asthma, when following the protocol.

First, one must determine their BOLT (Body Oxygen Level Test) score. To do this, take a normal breath through your nose, followed by a normal breath out. Pinch your nose and time how long it is, until you feel the first sign that you need to take a breath. The number of seconds, determines your BOLT score.

Next, breathe through your nose and not your mouth. Mouth breathing caters to asthma is several ways. Air taken in through the mouth, is not filtered of airborne particles, germs and bacteria. The mouth is not as effective as the nose, in conditioning air to the correct temperature and humidity prior to entering the lungs. The mouth provides a larger space to breathe through than the nose—thus the breathing volume will be higher, causing excess carbon dioxide to be expelled from the lungs. Carbon dioxide is a natural opener of the smooth muscle in the airways. Losing carbon dioxide, causes asthma airways to narrow even more. Mouth breathing does not allow us to benefit from nasal nitric oxide, which supports the lung's defense capabilities. With these combined factors working against mouth breathing, together they play a significant role in the exacerbation of asthma symptoms.

Up next, is the breathe tight to breathe right exercise. Place one hand on your diaphragm, and the other on your chest. Now breathe in through your nose, ensuring that the oxygen makes it to your diaphragm first—then into your chest. The goal is to reach a point where you can take a small inhale—which gets to your diaphragm—and then exhale. Practice this exercise for ten minutes a day. Take a break if you need to..

Lastly, practice breath holds. Take a small breath in and out of your nose, holding your breath and walking for 10 to 15 paces. Discontinue walking, and release your nose, while continuing to breathe in and out of your nose. Wait for 30 to 60 seconds, and repeat. Continue to walk while holding your breath for 10 to 15 steps, followed by resting with nasal breathing from 30 to 60 seconds. If your symptoms are mild, you may hold your breath for more than 10 to 15 steps. Do this for 10 minutes. This is important to warm up to, in order to avoid exercise induced asthma. Next, begin working out with only nasal breathing. If you feel as though you need to breathe through your mouth, slow down. It will take a little bit for your body to adjust.

Once you get your BOLT score to 40, you will no longer experience the symptoms of exercise induced asthma. While you can try this on your own, I do recommend at least reading the book for yourself, and/or setting up an appointment with someone who is trained in this method.

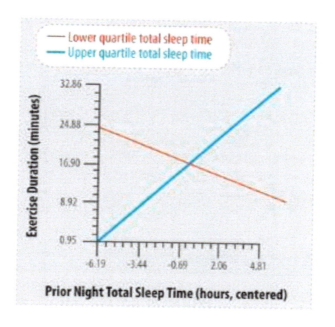

The Journal of Clinical Sleep Medicine performed a study to examine the effect that sleep has on workouts. Results of the study provide new insight into the relationship between exercise and sleep. The structure of the daily actigraphy, sleep, and exercise log data were utilized and collected for over sixteen weeks, for a unique perspective on the daily relationships between these variables in participants'

home environment over many nights. They found that exercise during the day was not associated with sleep during the corresponding night. However, sleep at night did predict the next day's exercise. Specifically, coefficients from the HLM model indicate that for every 30-minute increase in sleep onset latency above the individual's own average value, there was a one minute decrease in next day exercise duration. For shorter sleepers, there was a stronger relationship between poor sleep and decreased next day exercise duration.

HRV monitoring is a great tool that allows the coach to have important conversations about what's going on at home and in the athlete's life, in order to help athletes get the most out of their training. Oftentimes, HRV monitoring leads to discussions about the importance of getting more sleep, drinking less alcohol, and other behaviors that impact performance.

A university coach that I know, used this technology when the members of her soccer team suffered from six ACL injuries in one season. The coach implemented HRV monitoring during the following season with the same team, leading to an ACL injury free season. This anecdote illustrates the benefits of HRV monitoring. Through gathering heart rate data, coaches can prevent injuries by listening to the signals being sent by their athletes' bodies. The data allows us to detect an athlete's predisposition to hard physical training, dehydration, and other factors which affect recovery, and lead to injuries and other unwanted consequences. Athletes have not only been hurt, but have even died because they trained when their bodies were not ready. As coaches, it's our duty to take all necessary precautions to keep athletes healthy.

We once we had a college athlete who did not recover as well as the rest of the athlete in his group. The first time this happened, I let him take the day off from training to stretch, work on core, and perfect technique. The second time it happened, I asked him what was going on in his life outside of the gym. He claimed that nothing was bothering him, but I told him that his recovery data suggested otherwise. I told him that either something was going on or he needed to be examined for genetic anomalies which may have been hindering his recovery. He then revealed to me that he frequently drank alcohol, and got little sleep. We talked about the negative effects that those behaviors had on his body and the ways they prevented him from achieving his goals. HRV monitoring allowed us to discover the problem and come to a mutual understanding. Once we had this conversation, the athlete's behavior changed, and he went on to achieve his goals.

Without the HRV data, we risked learning about the issues only after he was injured, or worse. If we hadn't discovered the problems early on in the training process, he never would have achieved his goals. This is a prime example of why we monitor our athletes. There is a lot on the line, not only with their careers—but also with their health.

Find an HRV monitoring system that you like. Make sure that it has great reviews, and is easy for your athletes to use. We recommend getting a system where you can track all of your athletes in one place. This allows you to track more efficiently and quickly see where your athletes are at. For those who work in the private sector, this will allow you to monitor your athletes when they leave for college, or back to their pro team. Contacting them when they are not doing well will not only set you apart from the competition, but will deepen your relationship with your athletes. People need to feel cared for, and attended to. It's important that they know you care about their wellbeing.

Step 7: Re Test and Modifications.

DM ATHLETICS TRAINING PYRAMID

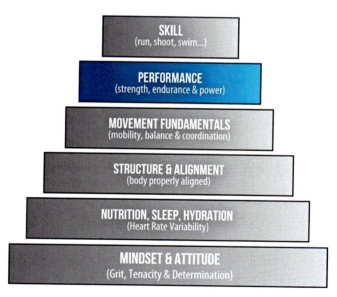

After the program is in place and athletes have begun training, we check their results on a monthly basis--or however often their program calls for it. We examine our athletes' posture and mobility to make sure they are improving. We also test their vertical jump, speed, and agility, to make sure those metrics are improving as well. We've found that our athletes get excited when they improve in any category, and it is extremely rewarding for us as coaches.

> "If you can't measure it, you can't improve it."
> Peter Drucker

Measuring results is vital to making sure that athletes progress toward their goals. Coaches need hard data to verify athletic improvement; judging performance on the way things "look" or "feel" is subjective and leaves athletes wondering about their progress. However, coaches can review data-based results with their athletes to measure progress and determine if the program requires any changes.

The greatest benefit of regularly testing athletes, is that it demonstrates where they are compared to where they were when they started. It also provides the coach with rationale for making certain program changes to help athletes achieve their goals; for instance, a coach might recommend additional food consumption, more rest, a change in the program, or something else.

Furthermore, when athletes can see how much they have improved and can also see where they ought to be for upcoming tests, they maintain a sense of excitement and begin to see their coach as a vital component of their progression in the sport. When athletes don't see measurable results, on the other hand, they are left wondering whether they have improved. This uncertainty hinders athletes' enthusiasm for training and makes it likely that they will switch coaches and find someone else to help them, or even stop training altogether —a lesson that we've learned the hard way.

Athletes should always seek coaches who measure results, because results drive performance. Imagine working hard at anything you care about and not having any proof that you are getting better. Many of us fall into the mindset that we are putting time and money toward this improving—so it must be getting better. The truth is however, that only if you are consistently tracking where you are, will you know if you are improving in any area.

I've witnessed coaches fudging the numbers, and finding ways to make their athlete's results look better than they actually are. This has more to do with ego, and the desire to be esteemed in a certain way by their athletes and community. They may even have a higher up that they must answer to. These are larger issues which need to be unpacked, but to their own fault, we want to see our athletes improve so much that we get too excited and hit the stop watch faster than we should. Or we help them on lifts, without realizing we are doing so. It's difficult to catch yourself in these moments but it is a discipline that everyone must improve on.

To time our runs, we prefer, to use electric timers because it takes the human factor out of it. Having an unbiased machine timing athletes, will give you results that will not be compromised. Now that being said, the problem which arises with electric timers, is that they are going to be slower than hand time from about two tenths to three tenths of a second. Athletes will compare themselves to kids their age, and even professionals or kids that perform at the NFL combine. Their numbers will be nowhere close because the kids their age are using handheld timers, and at the NFL combine the start of the 40-yard dash is still done by hand. The clock stops by a machine but it still is a tenth or two faster than a laser timer.

In order to give them hand times, we utilize a stopwatch along with the laser timer. We do this to show what their times are compared to what the laser time is showing, and also what other kids their age across the country are doing. It's a small detail which makes a big difference in the confidence of young athletes.

When we max out for lifts, we try not to touch the bar at all so they know that they've completed the lift on their own. That shouldn't be mistaken to read as us leaving them on their own. We stay as close as we can to the bar and their body, so if and when they do need a spot, we are able to do it quickly. It takes some practice, but when you do this during normal lifts when they are not maxing out, it will become easy. The spotting technique will be different for each lift, but for those who have been coaching for some time, you likely have this down. For those who are new to coaching, find someone you trust, that you can ask to help you. This is a critical part of being a coach--making sure that your athletes are safe while they are lifting weights.

Continuing athletes on their training program after they have gained amazing, measurable results can be difficult because at that point, they must work extremely hard to make only small improvements. This is mentally challenging because people are wired to seek big rewards and gain them quickly. At our facility, however, we try our best to celebrate small victories and improvements and show our athletes that small, continuous improvement always wins in the end.

Michael Jordan increased his vertical jump by ten inches over the course of five years, during his time as a professional athlete. That is a substantial gain, but when you average it out, it comes down to just two inches each year. Most people do not have the willpower to continue training when things are not improving as quickly as they like, even though—as Michael Jordan demonstrates—small, measured improvements add up to large gains. Athletes need to understand that the greatest results will happen during the first year of training. Once the body adapts to training, the measured results will slow, and everyone's ability to improve has a limit.

In order to continue improving, athletes need to focus on the constant grind, and acknowledge small improvements. At the elite level, for instance, small improvements can have huge rewards for athletes. Being a tenth of a second faster, jumping a couple of inches higher, or changing direction just a little more quickly than an opponent, are huge advantages in competition. These advantages can make the difference between making plays and not making them—and, ultimately, can mean the difference between playing and being out of a job.

Step 8: Mindset

DM ATHLETICS TRAINING PYRAMID

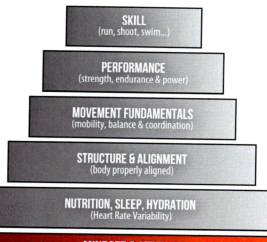

When it comes to performance, mindset is the most vital component. Simply getting athletes to give every workout everything they've got, will produce great results, no matter which school of training you follow. Oftentimes this component gets overlooked, especially these days when there are so many different studies and research which is done, to see what works best to improve athletic performance. We get caught in the details so much so, that we fail to bring the energy, enthusiasm and attitude to each session we spend with our athletes. As a result, their conditioning fails to drive their emotions like a game does.

For athletes coming off of an injury, the mental component is vital. Having returned from multiple injuries in my career, I know how uncomfortable it can be to get back on the field after sitting out for seven months or longer. You're tentative and worried about not getting hurt again. The best thing to do is to ease your way back in. Maybe starting with doing all the drills that do not require contact and then slowly adding contact drills back in. The goal here, is to build confidence in the athlete as they transition back to playing.

I remember coaches would yell at me or even put me down, for being scared to go full speed and hit someone. I found these experiences to be unhelpful. As an athlete and competitor, there is nothing you want to do more, than get back to normal. Put downs and insults do nothing but break down the relationship between a coach and an athlete. Although I knew that I was tough and capable of defending myself, it's important to note that this mentality only creates more issues. It's easy for some coaches to believe that they are doing the right thing because they are pushing you; however, study after study proves that this style of motivation is counterproductive.

The best way I've found to motivate athletes, is to bring as much energy as you possibly can to every workout, practice and game. I'm not talking about the false form of energy where some coaches will just yell all the time. Your players are not stupid, and can sense when something is forced and not authentic. What I recommend, is that you bring as much excitement and enthusiasm to everything you do with your team. It's difficult to do this day in and day out, but you'll be able to execute this when you really love what you do. It's too difficult to bring excitement and enthusiasm to something you do not love. Add to that a couple of losses, and it becomes even harder. If you're not in it because you love it, then you will not give your best effort day in and day out in order to help your athletes be their best.

I played defensive line in high school and college, and the most difficult thing we had to do is to take on a double team block by two three-hundred (sometimes more) pound guys. I had been thrown on the ground on several occasions, until I learned the main component required for success fighting this block; mindset! I grew up in a place where I was physically and mentally tested on a regular basis by other boys, my siblings, cousins and parents. As a result, I learned that to be the most effective in a physical altercation, you need to let go of the thinking part of your brain, and turn on the attack portion, which heightens your focus and releases more energy for you to fight. Only after I did this, was I was finally able to beat this block. That is the same attitude you and your athletes need to bring to your workout daily, because that is the attitude which will give you the best chance for success during competition.

Tom Waits said, "The way you do anything is the way you do everything". During training sessions we need to bring out the mindset that our athletes need in order to be successful. If a person hasn't been in a situation where they've experienced this, it will be difficult for them to understand. It is documented in *The Talent Code* by Daniel Coyle, the best coaches were once players themselves that failed to reach their ultimate goal. The reason is because they have been through the fire, and realized what worked and what doesn't. In training sessions and practice, you push your athletes beyond their limit, so that when it is game time you can sit back and let them go.

Don't underestimate energy. If you want your athletes to have a lot of energy during the game, you need to bring the intensity to the weight room and at practice. When two teams are evenly matched, the determining factor will be which team plays with more energy or intensity. Now it is on us as coaches to control the energy level we bring, because the athletes will feed off of us. We are in charge. It does not work the other way around. The most important thing is to keep a pulse on where the energy level is for the team. There are always highs and lows. The key is that when we notice the energy level coming down, we need to be doing something to raise it back up. The most successful thing we've found is doing something active to change the energy of not only the athletes, but the coaches. Perhaps creating some kind of competition, to change things up and regain their focus.

I've listened in, as coaches tell their athletes to bring more energy. I know what they're trying to do, but when you do this, you are down playing your role as the coach. As the coach, we are the leader--not the other way around. You need to realize that athletes will start to match our energy level and the way we think and talk. It doesn't matter if they agree with us or not. The athletes will take on the personality of their coach. Make it positive, focused and enthusiastic. This will put your athletes in the best position to be successful.

Most people only think of talent when it comes to sports—even the experts. Sports is actually where the whole idea of being "a natural" was born. "A natural" is someone who moves, looks, and is an athlete without having to work hard. Since so many people believe in natural talent, many professional coaches and scouts only look for naturals--paying huge amounts of money to recruit these individuals.

Unfortunately, many coaches look back with frustration when they finally realize that some of the most talented athletes, the "naturals", never really achieved great success. Why aren't these talented athletes successful? The real reason is that these athletes didn't have the correct mindset.

In her book, *Mindset,* Carol S. Dweck, Ph.D., talks about two different mindsets that athletes have about their abilities and talents. We touched on this earlier, in one of the first chapters. Athletes with a fixed mindset feel that their abilities and talents are fixed. They have what they have, and that is it. With a fixed mindset, athletes often become so preoccupied with looking and being talented that they don't realize their full potential.

The other mindset is of course, the growth mindset. Athletes with this mindset think of their abilities and talents as things they're able to grow and develop. They realize that with practice, instruction, and effort, they can realize their full potential. The growth mindset recognizes talent, but it focuses on developing and building on talent, instead of displaying talent and trying to simply coast along to success.

The Fixed Mindset

Athletes with a fixed mindset believe that their intelligence and skills are already determined and can't be changed. This mindset often results in emotional athletes who continually compare themselves to others. The result is a fearful, rigid athlete that has limited their potential.

Athletes with a fixed mindset usually feel that:
- Challenges should be avoided
- People are born with talent
- Perseverance doesn't help
- Challenges may show off a lack of skill
- If individuals have to work hard, it's because they aren't good enough
- Effort isn't really needed
- If failure occurs, it's the fault of someone else
- Feedback is something to take personally

The Growth Mindset

When athletes have a growth mindset, they believe that they can improve and develop their intelligence and skills. This means they're able to both win and lose gracefully, and they're also able to enjoy and share the successes of other athletes. This mindset results in open minded, hardworking, calm athletes who are coachable--making them capable of reaching their full potential.

Athletes with a growth mindset think that:
- They can improve upon their skills
- Skills are a result of hard work
- Challenges offer a chance to test themselves
- Mastery comes from effort
- They should embrace challenges
- They can learn from feedback
- Setbacks offer opportunities to learn
- Setbacks can be a wakeup call
- Feedback can be used to help find areas that can be improved upon
- Effort is an essential trait

Fixed vs. Growth Mindset–What That Means for Coaches

Coaches are in a unique position that allows them to help mold an athlete's mind, regardless of their age. Because they are privy to this opportunity, it's essential that coaches work with each athlete to specifically develop the growth mindset. This often comes down to the coach's values and how they praise their athletes.

Some of the best athletes are those which make the most mistakes. Oftentimes, they're unafraid of making mistakes. They realize that mistakes allow them to learn something, further helping them to achieve a higher level in the game. While this is a result of their own mindset, there's also a direct correlation between this and the type of praise which comes from the coaches.

It's common to see parents, trainers, and coaches who believe that winning is the only thing that matters. Unfortunately, this sets up athletes to have a fixed mindset. Athletes begin to play to avoid mistakes, instead of expressing their personality by trying things that may not be in their comfort zone. Taking a chance and making a mistake, teaches them what does and doesn't work, helping to increase their skill faster than those who work simply to avoid mistakes. Athletes with a growth mindset grow, achieve, and learn far more than individuals with fixed mindset.

Through my lifetime involvement in sports, I've been able to witness both ends of the spectrum, and I can guarantee that only athletes who have or adopt the growth mindset, have a chance of realizing their full potential. Injury always plays a role, and can derail anyone from achieving their goal. Within the growth mindset group, there is one aspect that I have come to notice which seems to separate the all-time best, and the rest of the pack. That mindset is what I like to call the attack mindset. In studying Michael Jordan, Muhammad Ali, Kobe Bryant, and several others who are considered the best to ever perform in their fields, I found this attack mindset. It's a mindset where they would not be denied, and did whatever it took to achieve their goals.

Let's dive into attack. When a Lion attacks its prey it brings everything it has from power, speed, and instincts--tapping into a place which brings out everything the Lion needs in order to make that kill. The reason why the Lion does this, is because it needs to eat. That is the why. Their approach is also simple; by any means necessary. The same can be said of Michael Jordan when he was with the Chicago Bulls. He had a burning desire to be the best. He achieved it by any means necessary.

Jordan started lifting heavy weights during the season, which was unheard of for basketball athletes. He admittedly disliked doing it, but realized that he needed to do so, if he wanted to accomplish his goals. Ali came up with his own tactics in the ring to defeat Forman. Taking hits is still not good for you no matter what level of boxing--but he used this to win the title back. Kobe rebranded himself the "Black Mamba", and went on to win two more championships.

Studies show that in an hour, we are only present on average, 10% of the time, 50% of the time we are thinking about a time in the future, and 40% of the time we are thinking about the past. When you attack something, you are 100% in the present moment.

Your brain will release more testosterone and cortisol to help in your efforts.

When you attack, you are no longer thinking—you are moving. You've got your eye on the outcome, but are focused on overcoming the obstacle which is currently in your way. When you attack, you become the hunter and your opponent becomes the hunted. When we get our athletes to attack, they no longer think about their prior injuries and how they feel, but they just go.

While your brain is in attack mode, your fears subside. Your fear of losing, making mistakes and even of death, in cases of combat fighters and other contact sport athletes, go away. This allows athletes to be more effective and perform at a higher level. It has been documented that the most productive fighter pilots and soldiers are the ones who are able to overcome this fear and do what is required of them. We use our brains and think critically, analyzing things around us, which is crucial--but when it comes to performing at your highest level, this will prevent you from reacting as quickly, and will slow your performance.

When the mind is completely focused, we respond quicker. Athletes continue to push themselves even more, reaching a point where they are in a flow. They have a feel for the game, and are able to make plays with less effort. Some call this "in the zone" or "flow" or runners might call it "second wind". It only occurs when athletes push themselves over a long period of time. That being said, it doesn't just happen--you need to bring your best effort and energy; day in and day out.

I vividly remember certain games in college where I achieved this flow state. I didn't try harder, yet things just happened. I made plays all over the field, with little to no effort. It was extremely fun but I never mastered competing every practice and every game in this state. The reason I believe I was not able to do so is that I was in fact, trying too hard. Sometimes when you push too hard, you reach a point where you begin working against yourself. There is a delicate balance between working hard and achieving flow, and pushing too hard where you make it impossible to achieve this state. Making practice fun and competitive, is one way which helps athletes to experience flow.

In college and especially in the professional level, athletics are big business. Some coaches take the same approach to practice, as they would a business meeting. The issue with this is that athletes need to be engaged, in order to get the best out of them. Boring practices which fail to foster enjoyment, ends up resulting in less engaged athletes, and producing bad results.

Now for us coaches, how can we facilitate this type of attitude throughout our team? Keep your team and athletes focused on their currently activity. If you are in a workout, focus on them attacking the workout and doing their absolute best in everything they do. When you are in practice, attack each drill with everything you have. When they get to the game, face each play head-on, with every ounce they have in their bodies. Only once you can create a single minded focus for your athlete, will they be able to perform their best.

The next thing you can do is create a fight mantra that they can say, to remind them to be strong and focused. This is not normal for people, but extremely powerful for teams that do use it. The New Zealand Rugby team performs the Haka before they play. Not only does this prepare them for their upcoming match but strengthens the relationship between everyone on their team. During World War 2, a battalion of Japanese Americans used the saying "Go fo Brok!" to motivate themselves and they were extremely successful in battle. Go for broke means to give it your all. The Tongan rugby team has a saying, "Mate Ma'a Tonga" (Die for Tonga), which is used for the same purpose. This saying has a deeper meaning because not only are they willing to die for their country, but also their family members and their brothers that they are fighting with on the field. If this is uncomfortable, getting your athletes to yell when they hit their opponent actually helps to release more power into that action. Just like martial arts or boxing, your breath will help you if you use it. In basketball, you can have something that triggers your athletes to play hard when they get on defense. Some guys slap the floor to get them to focus.

Each expression, chant, or dance, prepares each person for battle--leading them right into the attack mindset. The power of the group is dependent on how prepared each individual is, for the task at hand. When this mantra is repeated throughout practice and games, it will do nothing but help in your effort to create a singular focus while bringing the best out of each athlete. If you notice with all these sayings; the athlete is focusing on something bigger than just themselves. When they can remind themselves that their effort will have a direct correlation with the end goal, it will motivate people to keep pushing themselves.

You cannot just copy a saying and apply it to your team. One powerful thing you can do is to put the seniors or captains in charge of coming up with a battle mantra. This will put ownership on the leaders to come up with something their teammates can buy into, and they will take ownership of it. When coaches try to force this upon a team, sometimes it works, but most often, you do not get the buy in you need to make it successful—let your athletes come up with it.

Conclusion

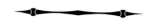

I hope that our training method will help many more athletes achieve their goals, stay healthy, and extend their careers. We have helped our athletes achieve amazing results that improved their performance, and also helped our athletes avoid any non-contact injuries. We hope you will adopt the method for yourself or your team so that you can give yourself or your athletes the chance to achieve the success that they—and you—deserve.

I know that there is a lot of information and there is more out there that I could have probably added to this. In fact, I am researching some things right now that have promise to be included in the next book I write; but for now, here is what we have. We will always research and study ways we can improve the results we get for our athletes and ways for them to stay healthy as long as they play. If you have any ideas how we can improve what we do, please reach out to us and let us know. We are totally open to experimenting and trying new things to see what works best.

My favorite coach of all time is John Wooden. He won 10 NCAA basketball championships in 12 years. If the rules at the time allowed freshmen to play, he probably would have won at least 11 out of 12 years because Kareem Abdul Jabbar had to sit his Freshman season even though he was the best player in the country. Coach Wooden always tried new things, even after he already won his 8th and 9th championship. If it didn't work—he would just scratch it but if it did—it made his team better and more competitive, and gave his athletes a better chance to be successful. That is what we also strive to do on a daily basis: find out what works best for our athletes so they can have the best chances for success in their sport and in life.

More than 80% of Coach Wooden's athletes went on to be successful outside of basketball. This is a far larger percentage than any university in the world, and that is including Ivy League schools or any coach that has ever coached. The reason is that his pyramid of success was not only meant to help his athletes to be successful on the court, but in life after their basketball careers were over. I truly believe sports teach you a lot but we have to be open to suggestions and what our experiences and coaches are teaching us while we play.

It is our main goal to not only help athletes play at their best and avoid injuries, but to be extremely successful after they get done with playing their sport. We know that we only have a short time with our athletes depending on how far they go in their careers. We strive to make every opportunity that we connect with them positive and inspiring. Not only to push through the difficult times that training present but to keep an open mind to doing things differently because there will always be a better way to do something. Whether it is a technique in their running or lifting, breathing properly and even small things like getting the right amount of quality sleep. All these factors not only play an important role in helping with athletic performance but with performance in anything that they choose to do after their athletic career is over.

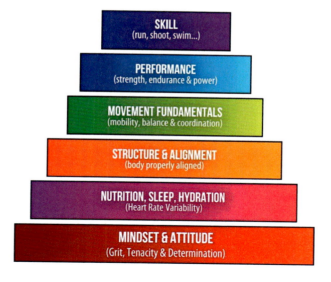

I just got done reading Tom Brady's book, The TB12 Method, and he recognizes the fact that he was not athletically gifted and had to work extremely hard in high school and in college to get playing time. When he got to the NFL, he knew how important the small things were in order for him to compete at his best. I do not think there is another athlete in the world that currently puts in the time dedication to every aspect for his training and recovery as Tom Brady and that is why he is able to perform at such a high level into his 40's. He sleeps 9 hours a night, drinks tons of water, eats the right food, works extremely hard and does every little thing he possibly can to gain a competitive edge. So many of the concepts that we covered in this book is embodied by him, which stresses how important these fundamental blocks are to performing at a high level.

First and foremost, his mindset, focus and attitude is amazing. That is the fundamental portion of our performance pyramid. Next is the attention to his sleep, hydration, nutrition is unmatched, which is the HRV block of our pyramid. His workouts consist of what he calls pliability, which can fit into the structure of our performance pyramid. I am not totally sure of its effectiveness but I am open to learning and trying it at some point in the future. I have seen some videos of Tom Brady training and they work on some movement fundamentals, which fits into the movement section of our pyramid. His movement is still really poor. I know that we can help him improve this to a greater extent. They do their own performance metrics in their training which is the performance part of the pyramid and he works on his skills daily to cover that portion.

Michael Jordan had an amazing mindset when it came to competition. Like Brady, Jordan experienced a failure in high school that really drove him to work extremely hard and prove that he deserved a spot on the varsity team the next season. It stayed with Michael so much so that during his Hall of Fame speech, he told his high school coach that he made a mistake by cutting him his sophomore season.

Next his trainer, Tim Grover, would have Michael drinking a ton of water and eating the right kinds of foods so he would play at his best. Michael from what report say did not sleep much at night but would nap before night games. This is one area that Michael could have improved but he did everything else right. His trainer would utilize a form of Muscle Activation work that would work on Michael's structure along with movement fundamentals to make sure he didn't lose any range of motion while he got bigger and stronger from his workout program. Finally, like Brady, Michael would outwork everyone when it came to basketball skills.

J.J. Wyatt has an incredible mindset and is able to push himself far beyond what his competition is willing to. J.J. like Brady and Jordan did not have it easy in high school. He barely got recruited to play football in college and figured out that he had to work extremely hard to get playing time anywhere. He walked on at Wisconsin where he earned a scholarship and became a first round draft pick. It took Wyatt a couple years to become a pro bowl player and now he is arguably the best to have ever done it at his position.

While studying his workout plan and his approach to the game I was not surprised to see so many of the concepts we covered in this book covered. Obviously his mindset is solid. When it came to his HRV, Wyatt sleeps 10 hours a night, drinks tons of water and follows a strict nutrition plan. Wyatt also works on his movement daily to make sure he doesn't lose any range of motion in his hips, shoulders, legs and so forth. Wyatt can easily squat so his glutes can touch his ankles without losing proper position. It is amazing for someone his size so I know movement is something he works on daily. Wyatt also lifts weights and runs like a normal strength and conditioning program. From everything I read and watched, I don't know if he works on his structure, which is why he is dealing with some back issues at the moment but this method would help him overcome that.

I can go on and on about examples of great athletes that execute these things like Usain Bolt, Michael Phelps, Serena Williams, Roger Federer, Lionel Messi, Muhammad Ali, Floyd Mayweather, Kobe

Bryant, LeBron James and so forth. Their lives consist of following these concepts in some shape way or form. These athletes were not just extremely lucky. They might not have had all the pieces in our method in place but they have enough for them to perform at a high level. One thing that frustrates me when reading about these great athletes is that most people try to break it down to one thing. Either it could be genetics, mindset, work ethic and so on but in actuality it is a combination of several different factors which were all covered in this book. Somethings made more of a difference for some athletes than others because every athlete is unique and have their own needs to perform at a high level. Only with this method will you be able to figure out what is that thing you or your athlete needs most.

On the other end of the spectrum, there have been several athletes that have shown great promise but to go on and not fulfill their full potential. I am reminded of Robert Griffin III, Derrick Rose, Penny Hardaway, Bo Jackson and so forth. All these and many more athletes had something go wrong in their careers that prevented them from playing at their best as long as they would have liked. I am one hundred percent certain that something or a couple of things we went over in this book were missed and could have helped these guys continue or even come back and perform at a high level.

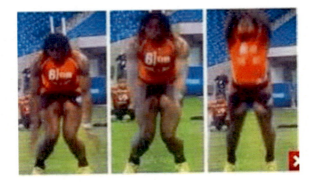

Here is a picture of Robert Griffin III, as you can see his knees are almost touching as he prepares to jump. This indicates that his structure is not in the best position for him to be successful. This is why he continues to have knee problems and if he does not address this issue, he will never play at the level of his rookie year.

In my experience I suffered a non-contact foot injury that indicates my structure was off. I also did not sleep 8 hours a night or ate the proper nutrition to give my body what it needed to perform at my best. After the injury, my movement was compromised in the weight room, on the field and most importantly while I played. Then my power, speed and ability to change direction declined to the point I had to sit the bench half way through my senior season. That caused my mindset and thoughts of myself to decline because I associated my identity with my ability to play football. Once that was gone, I had to rediscover who I am. I was depressed for a while but now I see clearly why I had to experience that.

It is never just one thing that happens but how it affects everything in your body. I had an injury that caused me to lose my ability to move like I use to, lifts weights and play football, which then made me lose my mindset. In getting athletes to get back to performing at a high level, each component needs attention. Some components of our performance pyramid might need more attention than others but only after a proper evaluation will we be able to know what those components are.

I think the most fascinating part to me in studying great athletes is after they achieved great success, like winning a couple championships, is how they continue to stick to their formula. Most people do not, because it's extremely hard and it's part of human nature to relax after you made a lot of money or reached the top of the mountain once. The goal of this book is to help more athletes reach their full potential. We broke it down step by step but as you can see, examples left by Tom Brady, Michael Jordan, J.J. Wyatt and other great athletes of that already showed us the way.

So let's review the steps to this method.

Step 1: Send your athlete to get a nutrition evaluation.

Step 2: Send your athlete to get a postural evaluation with some exercises they can do before workouts, practice and games that take 15 minutes or less. You can get a certification in different structural models but it is a long process so it is totally up to you.

Step 3: Movement Screening: Get certified in a movement screen. Test your athletes and find out their weaknesses. Then implement things into their program to improve their movement limitations.

Step 4: Test your athletes' performance. Get a baseline on their speed, agility, explosiveness and strength.

Step 5: Personalize their programs. With all the evaluations above and the testing, you will be able to easily individualize programs for your athletes. Even the programs you utilize now will be more effective by adding these components.

Step 6: HRV Monitoring. Pick a system you like and start tracking your athletes.

Step 7: Follow up Modification (Test again). Make sure that your athletes are improving. If they are not, it is a sign to change the program.

Step 8: Mindset – bring the right mindset to each workout and instill it into your athletes. Control the energy level during the workout and at practice. Make them feel like they are in a game by having high energy, creating competition but also maintaining focus throughout the workout and at practice.

This may seem to be a long process, but in actuality, this only adds 15 to 20 minutes to the workout. That time can be gained by just having the athletes come in 15 to 20 minutes early so you will not lose any actual time. The results you will gain by following this method are well worth the time spent on it.

Please do not think you can pick and choose between everything we have given you in this book. Yes, each individual thing will give you great results, but doing them all together will yield the best results for your athletes and your team—in terms of athletic performance and injury prevention.

The biggest obstacle that I have noticed is not from the extra time it takes to execute or track but from the willingness of coaches adopting something new. Most people get set in their ways and trying something new is uncomfortable, so they find ways to criticize it so they do not take any action that makes them uncomfortable. Also, some coaches feel threatened when something new comes out that contradicts the ways they have always done things. This is completely normal. In every field and every area of life, that is how some people choose to respond. For those who are uncertain about this, just try one suggestion. If it works out, try another one and move on from there. I spent over a decade figuring this out, so I know it works but I myself took it one step at a time until I got all the pieces together. I am still excited to learn new things and try it out because I am on a mission to provide the best training for athletes that this world has ever seen—but I know it will be one step at a time.

Feel free to contact me at dmathletics.com if you have any questions. Follow us on Facebook, Instagram and our Podcast which is the same title as this book. We will have athletes, coaches, authors of books mentioned here, scientist and so many guest on to help continue to improve our knowledge so join us in the movement. Please share this with friends, family and whoever you think will benefit from this information. Thank you and good luck!

Made in the USA
Lexington, KY
16 June 2018